Essential Oils

30 Recipes To Help You Lose Weight

Table of content

Introduction

That alarm is going off again, telling you it's time to get up and start another day. You can't hit the snooze button anymore, you have to get up and go, go, go. Get the work done, get the chores done, take care of the kids, get the errands done.

Your schedule is so full you don't have time to think about yourself.

And you notice the consequences of that. You have stress that seems to follow you around everywhere. You can't make the recipes you want to make or get to the gym like you used to, and your jeans just don't fit like they used to.

All in all, you want to make a change. A change that is going to last, and a change that is going to truly change your life. Something that's natural, because it doesn't do you any good to sacrifice on unhealthy things in life and use synthetics as your backup.

If you want to lose stress and lose weight the right way, you need to go about it the right way. Natural remedies are every bit as good as the synthetic ones when it comes to giving you the results you want, and I dare say they are even better in the long run because you don't have to worry that they are going to cause other side effects in your body.

But if they work so well, why don't you see them on all the advertisements like you do the synthetic things?

Think about it, if they were to manufacture synthetic items and not advertise them, they wouldn't sell. You don't have to advertise what is found in nature, and you can get the exact same results if you know how and when to use them. Which is what this book is going to do for you.

You will be equipped with the knowledge you need to make the right blends for the results you want, causing your stress and weight to melt away like you wouldn't believe is possible.

So are you ready to embrace a new you?

I bet you are...

So let's get started.

Chapter 1 – Weight and Stress: The Relationship Between the Two

In your mind, you are stressed from the life you live, and you blame your weight on the way you eat. You tell yourself you should go on a diet, or you should take those diet pills, or this, or that.

You stress about what you have to do in a day, and when you see yourself in the mirror or stand on the scale you stress all the more. Your life is becoming one giant blob of stress with you at the middle. Your weight is just the annoying bonus thing you have to worry about when you are lying in bed late at night.

I have something to tell you, and while it isn't going to fix all of your problems, it is going to give you a double benefit. How would you like to get rid of that stress... and lose that weight... all at the same time?

I know it sounds crazy, but you can.

You see, your stress level has a direct connection to your weight gain. This can happen in different ways, and it really doesn't matter how it happened in your situation, what matters is that it did, and you need to now fix it.

Emotional eating may be one of the factors that caused you to gain weight. You stress about what is going on down at the office, so you eat to take your mind off it. You eat because it feels good, you eat because you are happy, sad, bored... whatever.

The issue here isn't that you are eating, but that you eat when you are stressed, and it becomes your coping mechanism... thus causing you to gain the weight which in turn causes you to stress further.

Another thing happens when we are stressed. Our bodies release chemicals that cause us to hang onto the weight that we have. So no matter how many times you try to go on that diet, your body thinks you are in danger because of the stress hormones that are flowing around inside of it.

So, the natural response your body has to this situation is to hang onto the weight for all it can. So, when you spend months on a diet and maybe a certain level of exercise, you still see that your number stays the same on the scale. Or you can lose some for a little while, then it shoots back up again.

This causes more stress.

You can see there's a vicious cycle here, stress causing weight problems which are then causing you to stress once more.

You have to break out of this cycle the right way. You need to do it in a way that will last. Fad diets and diet pills only do so much, if you use them for a while, you are going to gain all of that weight back as soon as you get off of them. Think of them like band aids to the problem, when what you need is the solution.

There's good news!

The solution here lies in essential oils.

I know that sounds crazy right now, but let me show you why essential oils are going to help you lose the stress and the weight in your life, and why they will help you keep it off for good.

This isn't some elaborate plan that is designed to get you to purchase oils, this is a plan that has been designed to work. When you use it, you *are* going to be less stressed and you *are* going to lose weight. It's impossible not to.

So are you ready?

Chapter 2 – Why Essential Oils?

Before we get into the "how" of all this, I think you need to understand the "why". Success at anything is directly tied to your knowledge in why it works, because if you know why you don't be tempted to stray from the method when it gets harder.

That's right, there are going to be times when this is harder than you want it to be. One of the biggest mistakes people in general make about weight loss and stress reduction is the expectation that you are going to shrink to a size 2 and be on cloud 9 from the very start.

That's just not going to happen. I am presenting you with a method that is going to change your life, but it is going to take time. Just as your stress and weight crept up on you over the course of months or even years, getting rid of it is going to take a little while.

The good news is that it will come off much faster than it came on, because you have the help of these oils, and the knowledge you need to make it happen.

Why are essential oils so important for stress reduction and weight loss?

For starters, essential oils are natural. I firmly believe you will get better results using the natural method of anything than you would if you turned to the synthetics. Our bodies were designed to live in the natural world, so use what is in the natural world to take care of it.

No human is designed in a lab, so neither should the medication we need come out of a lab. Essential oils are every bit as effective as the synthetics, but they are natural, easier to get to, and much easier to mix into your day. All you need is a few oils, a bottle, and a warmer, and you're set.

Essential oils have stood the test of time

How many times have you seen a new diet land on the market? How many times have you tried this diet or that diet, and only got the same results? How many times have you heard of this thing that gets rid of your stress, or that thing that gets rid of your stress, but you crawl through life dealing with your stress?

Too many times, that's the answer.

Essential oils have been around for thousands of years. There are records of the ancient Egyptians using them, the Chinese, countless Middle Eastern countries, and the list goes on. They have been using them for all kinds of things for as long as history records, including: aches and pains, weight loss, stress reduction, spiritual enlightenment, and more.

They are around because they work. If they didn't they wouldn't have lasted until this modern day, where they are growing in popularity faster than a wildfire.

Once you see how this works for you, you will jump onto the plan, and start seeing the results for yourself.

Give me the reason essential oils will help with my stress

I can tell you time and time again that essential oils are going to help with your stress level, but unless I give you the "why", you aren't going to be any better off in your mind than you would be if I were to give you a pill.

The reason essential oils help you de-stress is because they work with your brain. Our brains are designed to use the smells of things around us to read signals and make decisions. We use this when we smell smoke, smell dinner burning, smell natural gas, and so on.

This truth can work the other way, however, when it comes to losing stress. There are certain plants out there that work directly with our brains to get rid of stress. They are found all over the world, and their oils are collected. If you use this oil, and blend with other oils in the same category, you are going to get a powerful mix of stress reduction.

If you then put this mix in a diffuser or an oil warmer, you are filling your home with this smell. This is going to work in your brain to relax you, calm you down, and get rid of that stress that seems to just want to hang on.

Makes sense, doesn't it?

Think of it as aroma therapy with the power tools you need for ultimate success.

But what about weight loss? Can I breathe in weight loss fumes?

The answer to that is both yes and no.

First, we can get the bad news out of the way. You can't plug in a blend of oils into your warmer and expect to lose weight just because you breathe that in, no.

But here's the good news. First off all, you are going to be a lot more relaxed, which is the lubricant you need to get that weight melted off of you. Secondly, you can blend oils that help suppress your appetite, and use these oils in your day to help you eat less and stay on track.

Then, there's the third reason of the oils that boost your metabolism, burning the fat off of you with half the amount of work it would take for you to do otherwise. If you combine these three reasons, you have the tools you need to easily lose weight.

Of course, you still need to eat right and exercise, but now you will lose the weight when you do this instead of your body hanging onto it as much as it can. Your body is going to want to lose the weight, which is going to cause you to shed pound faster than any diet pill ever let you.

The biggest benefits of all come with oils in two ways.

You may want to lose stress and weight, but if you use these oils, you are going to get a plethora of other benefits that just tag along for the ride. You will have fewer headaches, your immunity will go up, your pains and aches will subside.

And they smell fantastic... this is going to eliminate the need for you to have an air freshener in your home, cutting back on the amount of chemicals you're exposed to in your day.

With all of these benefits listed out, it's a lot better to ask, "Why not essential oils?"

Chapter 3 – Losing the Stress Essentially

Now that you have the science behind the matter, let's get started. I think you noticed from what I said in the last chapter that you need to get rid of that stress first if you want to lose weight easier, and I meant it.

So, let's focus on how you can lose that stress.

Here are the top 15 best blends to use for stress reduction:

The Get Away Blend

15 drops lavender

5 drops rose

5 drops vanilla

Mix oils together and place in your diffuser or warmer. Burn for a few hours in the room you are in, or scatter a few warmers throughout your house and have your success in every corner.

The Goddess Blend

15 drops chamomile

5 drops rosewood

5 drops lemongrass

Mix oils together and place in your diffuser or warmer. Burn for a few hours in the room you are in, or scatter a few warmers throughout your house and have your success in every corner.

The Mountain Cabin Blend

10 drops patchouli

5 drops vanilla

5 drops bergamot

5 drops lemongrass

5 drops cedar

Mix oils together and place in your diffuser or warmer. Burn for a few hours in the room you are in, or scatter a few warmers throughout your house and have your success in every corner.

The Seaside Bliss Blend

10 drops bergamot

10 drops cedar

10 drops tea tree

Mix oils together and place in your diffuser or warmer. Burn for a few hours in the room you are in, or scatter a few warmers throughout your house and have your success in every corner.

The Stress Buster Blend

10 drops jasmine

10 drops vanilla

10 drops geranium

Mix oils together and place in your diffuser or warmer. Burn for a few hours in the room you are in, or scatter a few warmers throughout your house and have your success in every corner.

The Roman Hide Away Blend

10 drops Roman Chamomile

15 drops frankincense

5 drops myrrh

Mix oils together and place in your diffuser or warmer. Burn for a few hours in the room you are in, or scatter a few warmers throughout your house and have your success in every corner.

The Wildflower Blend

10 drops lilac

10 drops lavender

10 drops lemongrass

5 drops tiger lily

Mix oils together and place in your diffuser or warmer. Burn for a few hours in the room you are in, or scatter a few warmers throughout your house and have your success in every corner.

The Hugs and Happiness Blend

10 drops vanilla

15 drops jasmine

5 drops lemongrass

5 drops geranium

Mix oils together and place in your diffuser or warmer. Burn for a few hours in the room you are in, or scatter a few warmers throughout your house and have your success in every corner.

The Starry Night

15 drops lemongrass

5 drops myrrh

5 drops marjoram

5 drops German chamomile

Mix oils together and place in your diffuser or warmer. Burn for a few hours in the room you are in, or scatter a few warmers throughout your house and have your success in every corner.

The Quiet Blend

15 drops bergamot

5 drops orange blossom

5 drops lemongrass

5 drops orange

Mix oils together and place in your diffuser or warmer. Burn for a few hours in the room you are in, or scatter a few warmers throughout your house and have your success in every corner.

Peace and Tranquility

15 drops peppermint

5 drops frankincense

5 drops patchouli

5 drops sage

5 drops lavender

Mix oils together and place in your diffuser or warmer. Burn for a few hours in the room you are in, or scatter a few warmers throughout your house and have your success in every corner.

Mountain Monks

15 drops sandalwood

10 drops valerian

10 drops cedar

5 drops vanilla

5 drops myrrh

Mix oils together and place in your diffuser or warmer. Burn for a few hours in the room you are in, or scatter a few warmers throughout your house and have your success in every corner.

Fairy's Harp Blend

10 drops rosewood

10 drops cedarwood

5 drops jasmine

5 drops lavender

5 drops geranium

Mix oils together and place in your diffuser or warmer. Burn for a few hours in the room you are in, or scatter a few warmers throughout your house and have your success in every corner.

Crickets and Sunsets

15 drops ylang ylang

5 drops cedar

5 drops pine

10 drops blood orange

5 drops lemongrass

Mix oils together and place in your diffuser or warmer. Burn for a few hours in the room you are in, or scatter a few warmers throughout your house and have your success in every corner.

Goodnight Moon Blend

10 drops valerian

10 drops geranium

5 drops peppermint

5 drops cedar

5 drops lemongrass

5 drops honeysuckle

Mix oils together and place in your diffuser or warmer. Burn for a few hours in the room you are in, or scatter a few warmers throughout your house and have your success in every corner.

Please note:

Essential oils are a very controversial subject when it comes to ingesting them. Some people say you shouldn't ever ingest them under any circumstance due to possible toxicity and overdose, but others claim that it's just fine so long as you dilute them well and only take recommended amounts.

I say it's up to you what you want to do, but if you do ingest, then please only take 1 or 2 drops in an entire day, and dilute those drops well when you use them.

Chapter 4 – Boosting the Following Weight Loss

Now that you feel light and airy as you should, it's time to get into the weight loss issue. You have what it takes to lose that weight easily now, so let's give you a boost in the right direction.

Remember that you still need to eat right and exercise, so the first thing you need to do is find a healthy eating plan that works for you. I'm not saying a diet plan that is going to restrict you, but a well balanced plan that is full of fruits, veggies, lean meats, and even the sweets that you crave from time to time.

Set yourself up for success, and you will enjoy that success in the long run. The more you plan for your life in 10 years, the more likely you will be to have that life in 10 years.

So find a diet plan you enjoy, and can stick with, then add onto that an exercise regime you can also stick with. One that gets your heartrate up for about half an hour a day, 4 or 5 days a week.

Once you have these things in place, it's time to start up the oil blends that are going to push your weight loss to the max in no time.

The Every Day Blend

15 drops grapefruit oil

10 drops lemon oil

5 drops peppermint oil

5 drops orange oil

Mix oils together and place in your diffuser or warmer. Burn for a few hours in the room you are in, or scatter a few warmers throughout your house and have your success in every corner.

The Holiday Blend

10 drops vanilla

10 drops peppermint

10 drops ginger

5 drops cinnamon

Mix oils together and place in your diffuser or warmer. Burn for a few hours in the room you are in, or scatter a few warmers throughout your house and have your success in every corner.

The Celebration Oils

15 drops vanilla oil

15 drops rose oil

5 drops argon oil

5 drops frankincense oil

Mix oils together and place in your diffuser or warmer. Burn for a few hours in the room you are in, or scatter a few warmers throughout your house and have your success in every corner.

The Weekend Blend

5 drops lilac oil

5 drops lemon oil

5 drops lime oil

5 drops orange oil

Mix oils together and place in your diffuser or warmer. Burn for a few hours in the room you are in, or scatter a few warmers throughout your house and have your success in every corner.

Company's Coming

10 drops vanilla oil

10 drops cinnamon bark

10 drops blood orange oil

10 drops nutmeg

10 drops ginger

10 drops orange

Mix oils together and place in your diffuser or warmer. Burn for a few hours in the room you are in, or scatter a few warmers throughout your house and have your success in every corner.

The Bad Day Blend

10 drops pine oil

10 drops lemon oil

10 drops peppermint oil

5 drops tea tree oil

Mix oils together and place in your diffuser or warmer. Burn for a few hours in the room you are in, or scatter a few warmers throughout your house and have your success in every corner.

The High Five Blend

10 drops grapefruit oil

5 drops cinnamon oil

5 drops bergamot

5 drops saffron

5 drops peppermint oil

Mix oils together and place in your diffuser or warmer. Burn for a few hours in the room you are in, or scatter a few warmers throughout your house and have your success in every corner.

The Kickstarter Tool

15 drops fennel

15 drops lemon

5 drops lemongrass

5 drops lavender

Mix oils together and place in your diffuser or warmer. Burn for a few hours in the room you are in, or scatter a few warmers throughout your house and have your success in every corner.

The Success Blend

15 drops patchouli

5 drops pine

5 drops balsam fir

5 drops lavender

Mix oils together and place in your diffuser or warmer. Burn for a few hours in the room you are in, or scatter a few warmers throughout your house and have your success in every corner.

The Fat Burner Deluxe

15 drops ocotea oil

5 drops tea tree oil

5 drops bergamot

5 drops cinnamon bark

Mix oils together and place in your diffuser or warmer. Burn for a few hours in the room you are in, or scatter a few warmers throughout your house and have your success in every corner.

The Powerhouse Blend

15 drops ginger

15 drops lemon oil

15 drops lime oil

Mix oils together and place in your diffuser or warmer. Burn for a few hours in the room you are in, or scatter a few warmers throughout your house and have your success in every corner.

The Catapult

10 drops ginger

10 drops black pepper

15 drops cedar wood

15 drops geranium

Mix oils together and place in your diffuser or warmer. Burn for a few hours in the room you are in, or scatter a few warmers throughout your house and have your success in every corner.

The Runner's Blend

15 drops nutmeg oil

15 drops ledum oil

15 drops balsam fir

15 drops black pepper

Mix oils together and place in your diffuser or warmer. Burn for a few hours in the room you are in, or scatter a few warmers throughout your house and have your success in every corner.

The Bikini Blend

15 drops grapefruit oil

5 drops copaiba

5 drops lavender

5 drops lime oil

Mix oils together and place in your diffuser or warmer. Burn for a few hours in the room you are in, or scatter a few warmers throughout your house and have your success in every corner.

The Athlete Blend

5 drops cinnamon

5 drops vanilla

5 drops ginger

5 drops peppermint

Mix oils together and place in your diffuser or warmer. Burn for a few hours in the room you are in, or scatter a few warmers throughout your house and have your success in every corner.

Please note:

Essential oils are a very controversial subject when it comes to ingesting them. Some people say you shouldn't ever ingest them under any circumstance due to possible toxicity and overdose, but others claim that it's just fine so long as you dilute them well and only take recommended amounts.

I say it's up to you what you want to do, but if you do ingest, then please only take 1 or 2 drops in an entire day, and dilute those drops well when you use them.

Dilution tips and carrier oils

For the oils you do decide to ingest, there are different ways you can do this that will help you get the best experience out of the occasion. If you don't care for the taste of the oil itself, and trust me, it's strong, then you can dilute it in 8 ounces of water.

That's 8 ounces of water per drop of oil you are using, so obviously if you are going to use 2 drops of oil you want to double the amount of water you use to dilute it with. You can, of course, use tea as well. This is a great way to get it inside without having to use the taste of the oil. If you use a peppermint tea or another kind of spice tea, the oil will blend with the flavor quite nicely.

If you are going to use the oils topically, you must blend them with a carrier oil so it doesn't harm your skin. You see, a lot of oils are very concentrated, so they may actually cause skin irritation if they are on your skin for any length of time. This is why it is important that you use the oils with another carrier oil.

The best carrier oils I have found are baby oil, coconut oil, and olive oil. Simply mix the oil of your choice with any of these oils, diluted to 1 drop per teaspoon of carrier oil, and apply to your skin this way.

That's it! With diligent use of these oils, you can get the results you want in no time at all! This is truly going to give you the results you are after in a matter of weeks, and they are going to be the results that will last.

Good luck!

Conclusion

There you have it, everything you need to know when it comes to losing the stress... and the weight... in your life. From what you saw in this book, the two tend to go hand in hand, and if you are able to control one of those aspects, you are going to be able to control the other.

I want you to remember one thing, this is a process. The oils are tried and true, and they are going to give you the results you want, but you have got to stick with it, and you need to be patient. If you are losing weight the right way, you will lose a little at a time, and see the big results you want over a period of time.

Weight loss that lasts is going to happen gradually, but once you do lose the weight, you aren't ever going to gain it back. Eyes on the prize is a good way to look at it, not to mention enjoying the journey.

No doubt you will be hooked on these oils from the start, so the more you practice, experiment, and blend, the more fun you will have in the method. You will find what you like the best, and you may even invent a few of your own.

The more you can incorporate these oils into your life, the richer your results are going to be. I know you can do it, and I know these oils are your ticket to success. All you have to do is be patient and stick with them.

So what are you waiting for? There's a relaxed, slimmer you inside, just waiting to get out and meet the world.

FREE Bonus Reminder

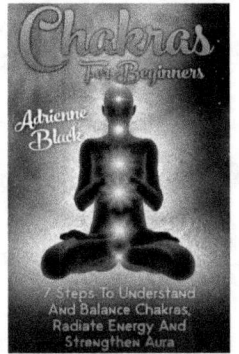

If you have not grabbed it yet, please go ahead and download your special bonus E book *"Chakras for Beginners. 7 Steps To Understand And Balance Chakras, Radiate Energy, And Strengthen Aura"*.

Simply Click the Button Below

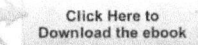

OR **Go to This Page**
http://lifehacksworld.com/free

BONUS #2: More Free & Discounted Books
Do you want to receive more Free & Discounted Books?
We have a mailing list where we send out our new Books when they go free or with a discount on Kindle. Click on the link below to sign up for Free & Discount Book Promotions.
=> Sign Up for Free & Discount Book Promotions <=

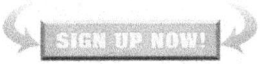

OR Go to this URL
http://zbit.ly/1WBb1Ek